SIMPLE

WEIGHT LOSS

SYSTEM™

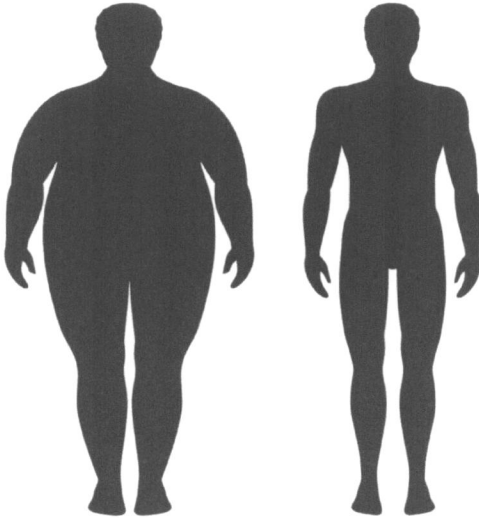

How To Easily Lose **22 Pounds** in Three Months!

Samuel F. Valle

October 2018: First Edition

Proofreader: Alex Solsbery

Copy-editor: Susan Ray

Composition: Karolina Kaiser (mobisfera.pl)

ISBN 978-83-65477-15-6

Contents

Introduction

Have you ever wondered how to drop twenty-two pounds* in the shortest time possible and then maintain your new weight? I'm sure you have, if you reached for this guide. I have good news for you—you can stop worrying about it at this moment, because the system described in this book works for everyone, without exception. All you need to do is read this book carefully and then stick to the system rigidly. If weight loss is a problem for you, it only means that your weight loss methods do not work. My weight loss system always works, so losing the extra pounds is not any problem for me. If I succeeded and other people around the world who have tried it are also successful, then you will succeed just as well. Remember: losing unnecessary pounds is really a simple thing. Embrace this confidence and apply the Simple Weight Loss System™ in your own life.

*Note: The United States has not adopted the metric system and refers to personal weight in pounds. Even though the UK utilizes the metric system, people still usually refer to their weight in stones and pounds (one stone equals 14 pounds, and one pound is 0.45 kilograms). Pounds will be used throughout the text, so if you are accustomed to the metric system, just remember one kilo is 2.2 pounds, and one pound is just a little less than half a kilo (0.45 kilograms).

1. My Story

A few years ago, I participated in an amateur MMA fight. It was supposed to last for three rounds of three minutes each, but it lasted only two rounds. I was not knocked out; my friend did not put any leverage or stranglehold on me, nothing like that. We just both felt totally physically exhausted. We were not even able to make it to the third round. The judge announced a draw, but I still felt like a big loser. Many years of working in front of the computer, a lack of exercise, and eating unhealthy food had done their jobs. I used to be a strong, energetic, athletic young man, and suddenly, at the age of twenty-nine, I was not able to move after going two three-minute rounds? This effort was so great for me that after the fight I threw up, then I slept fourteen hours straight. Immediately after waking, I felt like the most motivated person in the world to get rid of my unnecessary weight.

I weighed 190 pounds at the time at a height of six feet, and I immediately knew what my goal was—168 pounds. I had collected twenty-two pounds of fat due to my lack of exercise and high-calorie meals. My motivation was great, and the goal was clear and straightforward. The only question left was: How was I to do it?

First, I introduced more movement into my life. Unfortunately, the additional exercises had no significant effect on my weight loss. Nevertheless, I must admit that if you work at the computer about eight hours a day, then no matter which activity you start—walking, running, swimming, gym workout—they will all have a 100 percent positive effect on your body. Many people think that if they start running, they will burn fat and the weight will drop off by itself. When nothing changes and only their knee joints hurt, disappointment and discouragement sets in. They simply do not really know how to effectively remove fat from their body. Movement is only a healthy addition to the weight loss process, while the main key is the right diet. People who want to burn fat solely by running actually do not burn that many more calories than before, and they continue to supply too much fuel to their body. Sooner or later, anyone who is serious about losing weight will realize that the key to effective weight loss is the right modification of their current diet. In my experience, the effect of exercise on fat burning is around 20 percent, while the impact of diet is 80 percent.

2. Simple Weight Loss System™

2.1. Where does body fat come from?

Our bodies are the greatest biological factories in the world. Each day we deliver fuel to this factory, and each day we use it. Imagine that your factory consumes 2,600 calories per day, and you provide it with 3,400 calories. This intelligent system does not waste energy. Additional fuel is set aside in the warehouse so that in the event of a temporary break in delivery, the factory can continue to work smoothly by using energy from the warehouse. Adipose tissue (more commonly called body fat), which is what we are talking about, is the high-caloric part of our body that stores energy reserves. It forms when we systematically introduce an excessive amount of energy into the body in the form of sugars and fats.

2.2. Why is weight loss so difficult?

Losing body fat, first of all, requires changing our eating habits. Let's be honest, in most cases, if you're overweight, it's because you have bad eating habits. Changing habits causes people many problems, because the force by which habits affect people can be compared to the force of gravity. Man is attracted to perform a given activity (e.g., drinking sweet soda drinks) in the same way that an object is attracted to the Earth's surface. Fortunately, we have a system that allows us to overcome the force of gravity and launch a rocket into space. Just as a rocket burns the most fuel at the start, it takes a lot of effort to get started. As soon as you take off, I can assure you that the further you go, the easier it will get. Losing weight is difficult only because it requires changes in eating habits, and few people know how to go about this effectively.

2.3. What is the Simple Weight Loss System™ based on?

The Simple Weight Loss System™ is based on the basic principles of success: motivation, goal, and strategy. Motivation is the basic thing. If you do not really want to lose excess pounds and you're reading this book just because someone recommended it to you, I'm sorry but nothing will come out of it. For example, many bachelors seeking their future wife often declare that they "would like" to lose unnecessary pounds; however, deep down they really do not want to make the effort. How to get yourself motivated? Oftentimes, this cannot be achieved easily. Strong motivation must flow from inside. If you are not motivated, then no system will work for you. I assume that if you bought this book of your own choice, you have motivation and you only lack the goal and the strategy. If this is not the case, do not fool yourself because without strong motivation, you will give up after either a few days or a couple of weeks.

However, motivation is simply not enough. Without a goal, it's difficult to achieve success because we do not know what it is we are striving for. First, you have to weigh yourself, then look at the tables and determine for yourself exactly how many pounds you want to drop and in what amount of time. Let's assume that your goal is like mine: to lose twenty-two pounds in three months. This is a concrete and realistic goal. Losing twenty-two pounds in two days is an unrealistic goal. On the other hand, the loss of twenty-two pounds in five years is not a very ambitious goal. It is important that the goals you set for yourself are within your reach and realistic. Then you will have the conviction needed and you will find that the system works.

The strategy is like a cake recipe. We need to know exactly what to do in order to achieve a given goal. Many people think that a good strategy is the ideal recipe for success. This is not true. Strategy is only the third element of the entire puzzle. You must remember that the strong motivation flowing from inside, that is, the great strength that comes from "I want to lose weight" makes you do all the tasks with a smile on your face. However, strategy requires discipline and good organization on our part. If you miss these elements, I will help you introduce them into your new weight loss system that works in 99.99 percent of all cases.

The Simple Weight Loss System™ strategy is based on the gradual modification of your diet in the way that suits you best! I'm not kidding—you do not have to stick to broccoli and wash it down with water to make the system work. What you will eat depends only on your own choice; that's why my system supports you instead of imposing loads of restrictions upon what you will or will not eat.

2.4. Recommended pace of weight loss

Nutritionists report that the best weight loss rate is a little over two pounds per week, or about nine pounds per month. My experience shows that it's hard to keep this pace. Usually at the beginning the pace is high: about four pounds per week, and then in following weeks it gradually begins to fall to three pounds, two pounds, and as low as one pound per week. This is very helpful information when planning your *realistic goal*. In addition, notice that theoretically, we should be able to drop twenty-seven pounds in three months. But I set the bar at only twenty-two pounds in three months. Why do I lower the amount? I prefer to achieve success and have a positive attitude rather than to fail and then worry that it did not work out.

2.5. Where to begin?

First, I will try to help you understand the essence of the Simple Weight Loss System™ and then show how it is applied in practice. The beginning is always the toughest, so start by facing the following facts:

- current weight
- goal
- today's diet

Take note of these three things on a piece of paper. For example, my weight a few years ago was 190 pounds. My goal was to lose twenty-two pounds in three months, because I knew that it is unhealthy to lose more than nine pounds of body weight per month. My diet at that time looked more or less like this:

- In the morning: coffee + sandwich.
- Around noon: lunch ordered at work that usually included pizza or a piece of grilled chicken.
- At 5 p.m.: dinner of vegetables + a piece of meat.
- At 9 p.m.: supper of four sausage sandwiches.

That's how my whole day was. Somewhere in my diet I had smuggled in extra, unnecessary calories, but I did not know from where. To know exactly where I stood, I decided to balance the calories of the meals I ate. I called this stage: observation of current diet.

2.6. Your current diet

Diet is the way we eat. In reality, we are on a diet all our lives and not just for a few months. Diet does not simply mean a recipe for nutrition in order to lose weight. There are numerous types of diets that allow you to gain weight, strengthen immunity, detoxify the body, et cetera.

My diet before weight loss consisted of dishes that I decided to take a closer look at. A sandwich for breakfast is standard for me, but how many calories does it have? Four pieces of pizza at work was not enough to fill my stomach, but how many calories does such a meal contain? I decided to answer all these questions. I started browsing tables on the internet and writing down how many calories 100 grams of a certain food has and then estimated how many grams per day I ate. This is a job that you have to do yourself at this very moment. If you want to actually lose weight, immediately write on a piece of paper what you eat on each of your routine days. Then, next to each meal should be the number of calories. Try to be as accurate as possible, but remember that it is only a close estimate and that using home methods you will never be able to tell the exact number of calories you consume every day. However, remember that writing down the number of calories of specific meals is the only way you can control the amount of energy you deliver to your body yourself.

2.7. Weigh yourself regularly

The Simple Weight Loss System™ relies on modifying your diet at your own discretion. But I will try to give you a little help so that you do not make key mistakes that can lead to failure. Your actual weight is your only real measurement to go by. Forget about trying to use other measurements such as loose pants, a girl's compliment, or your impression after looking in the mirror. Only your weight will tell you the truth, so trust it. Weigh yourself regularly every week at the same time (e.g., always on Sunday morning). When you start to modify your diet and the first effects appear, the scale will start to smile at you, although in reality it is you who will be smiling. Nevertheless, regular weighing is not enough. You must record your weight and make graphs illustrating weight changes over time. There are many applications on the market available to measure and record your weight. In my case, the Excel program was very helpful. No matter what you use, the most important thing is that you weigh yourself regularly and record your weight. Do not do it too often or too rarely. It is best to weigh yourself once a week or once every two weeks.

2.8. Modifying your diet

The core of my method of losing unnecessary pounds is to modify your own diet at your own discretion. Note that this is the simplest and cheapest method. Why spend money on professional nutritionists if you are not an athlete or do not have serious health problems? Become your own dietitian today and pay yourself for what you do.

Many people make a mistake when modifying their diet. They drastically change their whole diet, all meals, the number of calories taken, meal composition, everything. Your body gets shocked, your mind rebels, and very soon after such an unsuccessful try, people return to their old eating habits. This is commonly known as the yo-yo effect. Avoid making the same mistake as everyone else. Realize that your body is used to your current diet, and it really likes it. If you drastically change your whole diet and instead of pizza you start to eat only cooked vegetables, do not be surprised later that it does not work. Which normal person is able to change everything in their life from one day to the next and not feel confused? For our bodies, diet is almost everything. Our bodies adapt to meal times, the amount of food eaten, and meal composition, and at fixed times secretes appropriate digestive enzymes. That's why I think—and this is confirmed by thousands of my satisfied customers—that the diet should be slowly and gradually modified so that your body, digestive system, and your mind have time to adapt to new conditions.

2.9. How to practically start modifying your diet

For my first diet modification, I started with limiting the number of calories consumed for the evening meal. Instead of four sandwiches, I started eating three, without changing their composition. Then after two weeks, I started eating two sandwiches, without changing their composition. After a month, instead of four sandwiches in the evening I ate one, and I felt full and satisfied. From my calculations, I could see that I had reduced the number of my calorie intake in the evening from 480 calories (4 x 120 calories) to 120 calories (1 x 120 calories). Note that I did not immediately stop eating four sandwiches in the evenings. The reasons are simple: my mind would feel that I had lost something, and my body would confirm it by feeling hungry. Instead, I gradually and slowly reduced the number of sandwiches so that, most of all, I wouldn't notice this change.

Decreasing the amount of food eaten is one very simple method. You can also change the composition of dishes. When changing the composition, it is important to keep the same principle as before. Try to cleverly "cheat" your mind so that it doesn't think that it is missing out on something. Instead of eating a fatty sausage, replace it with something else that you also *really* like to eat. Do not give up the sausage completely; eat it every other day or only on the weekend. But it is important to introduce the changes gradually and slowly. The most important thing is that you, or rather your mind, does not feel that it is a change for the worse, that you are missing something and don't feel good about it. Introduce new foods slowly and gradually without totally giving up the old but by reducing how often you eat it. For example, instead of eating sausage sandwiches, I started to eat turkey sandwiches. This way I eliminated a few unnecessary calories from the fat in the sausage. Reducing the number of calories in your diet will translate into weight reduction, and the effect is guaranteed.

The next step to reduce the number of unnecessary calories in your diet can be by replacing sweet soda drinks with pure water. Here, the same principle works. "Trick" your mind and your body. Instead of completely giving up sweet drinks, start to dilute them at a 3:1 ratio by mixing them with water. After two weeks, change the ratio to 2:1. After a further two weeks, change the ratio to 1:1. Then, introduce one glass of pure water daily, and so forth. All you need to do is diligently write down in your current diet notebook, your weight, and your diet modification experiments. However, remember that your aim is to lower calories in your diet and not increase them. Therefore, either reduce the volume of meals or replace high-calorie products with low-calorie ones. Everything you choose to eat should be something you like and that tastes good to you. At this point you start to control the right proportions for products because you care more about your health than before. The goal you set lets you know what you are aiming for. Therefore, your diet modifications are not a bother and a burden because you do it in a way that you continue to enjoy the food as before. If you have made a change in your diet that you are dissatisfied with, let it go and do not wear yourself for no reason. Having the attitude of *I do not like cauliflower, but I have to eat it because of my diet* is a key mistake. You are the boss in charge of your own diet, and you decide what you want and what you like to eat. The only tools helpful in the implementation of the weight loss process are your weight and the record of your current diet from which you gradually remove unnecessary calories.

2.10. Caloric balance

Note that our bodies strives for balance. It is the same in the case of food eaten and energy used. Your body strives for a zero-energy balance, which means that whatever food you consume, you burn. Therefore, after modifying your diet, you will surely come across a situation like the one described below.

Suppose that after changing your main meal of the day from a high-calorie pizza to a homemade dinner, your weight dropped by three pounds in two weeks. You are overjoyed with the results and continue eating the same way, thinking that in the next two weeks your weight will again drop by three pounds. However, this is not the case, and your weight only dropped by one pound. After the next two weeks, your weight remained the same instead of dropping. This is completely normal. Notice that if you have decreased the number of calories consumed from 3,200 to 3,000 and your weight has stopped dropping, then it is time to reduce the daily intake of calories from 3,000 to 2,800. In this way, you are able to get rid of unnecessary kilos without wreaking havoc on your body, which often happens with drastic types of diet, such as dropping to 1,000 calories per day. Please notice that the Simple Weight Loss System™ takes into account the fact that your estimation of consumed calories per day may be inaccurate. This does not matter that much, because the most important thing is that it is *you* who is now controlling what foods and what quantities you consume. You can see for yourself on the scale whether you are doing it right or wrong.

In addition, the Simple Weight Loss System™ gives you tools that will increase your motivation many times over. Believe me, if you see for yourself that your weight has dropped by a few pounds and you really got there on *your own*, then your self-esteem, confidence, and faith in the system will increase significantly. When you see your effort rewarded with a real result represented by a specific number on the scale, nothing will be able to stop you. Your current caloric balance may be 1,800, 2,000 calories, 2,500 calories, or 3,000 calories. But this is not that important because each of us is different and each of us leads a way of life that is more or less active. Remember that if your weight stays the same for more than a month, it means that your body will burn exactly as many calories as it gets, and you already know your caloric balance. If you want to burn more fat, you have to slightly modify your diet again and remove another 100 to 200 calories from it.

3. Simple Plan

3.1. Losing 22 pounds in 3 months

My first plan was pretty simple: I gradually modified my diet so that my weight would drop from 190 pounds to 168 pounds. I introduced changes to my diet every week because I know that the body adapts quickly to new conditions. I expected that after three months it would be harder for me to lose the next kilos, because my body would adapt and begin to like my new diet. I compiled the diet myself based on notes from the whole day, in which I convert every meal into calories. The most important aspect for me is the mental comfort and feeling happy about what I was eating. I did not want to get tired of my diet because I was eating something that I did not want to eat. I had a notebook in which I recorded my weekly body weight and the date. I kept a second notebook to prepare my own current diet and introduce my own modifications to reduce my consumption of calories.

Cheating yourself is not an option; if I eat more than I planned, I needed to admit to myself that I was being a dummy. I reduced the number of calories in my diet gradually by eating smaller meals (e.g., instead of four sandwiches, I would eat three) and slowly and gradually I replaced high-calorie products with lower calorie ones, while making sure that I enjoyed the taste. I did not take drastic steps. I started by reducing the number of calories by a maximum of 100 to 200 calories per day.

3.2. Implementing the plan

The plan is just theory, and its implementation is the most important. Therefore, from the moment of checking my body weight, calculating how many calories I eat a day, and applying a few changes that reduce the amount of food introduced to my body by 100 to 200 calories per day, I follow my plan. The first and second days were very easy. Problems usually appear after a longer time. But because the changes are not so radical, my body did not feel them too much. I can say, and many of my clients confirm the same, that following the Simple Weight Loss System™ is surprisingly easy and pleasant. I have moments when I want to eat something "forbidden," but then I take a look at my notes and decide to satisfy myself by eating something with fewer calories. I always support myself mentally with the words: "This is so delicious!" I do not want to break the rules I have set for myself because then my efforts would not make any sense.

Remember that it takes iron will to achieve your goal. You have to stick to your own plan from your notes, and because you have prepared it yourself, it is *much* easier than if it were prepared by someone else. The way the system works is that by preparing yourself a diet that is more suited to you and by introducing changes gradually and not radically, your body and your mind both feel satisfied. This is the best way to implement this simple plan of cutting unnecessary calories from your daily diet. If you reduce the number of calories in your plan and then eat more than you should have, it means that you do not really care about achieving your goal.

Below are my BEFORE and AFTER pictures using the Simple Weight Loss System™.

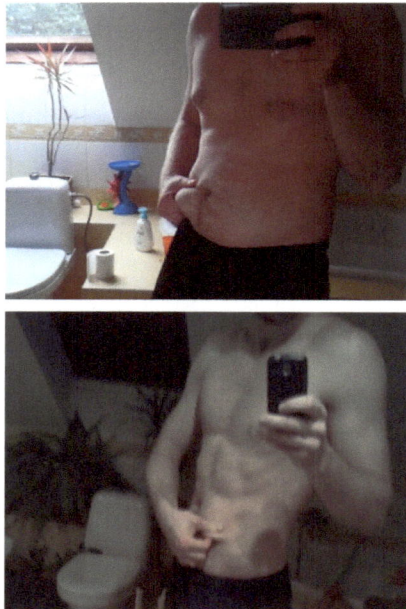

As you can see in the pictures, after three months of using my program, the effects are great. The amount of fat on my stomach decreased significantly. Dear reader, please also note that I am not an athlete, only an office worker. If you only want to lose excess weight, you've come to the right place. However, if you want to work on having a more athletic figure, this book is not enough.

3.3. Macro and micro elements

Although the Simple Weight Loss System™ has been designed to simplify the weight loss method to the maximum extent and achieve the best results in the shortest possible time without harming your health, at the same time, any dietitian will tell you that the macro and micro elements found in foods are very important for your health. The macro elements are proteins, fats, and carbohydrates, while the micro elements are vitamins and minerals. It is very important that your diet is not monotonous, that you make sure you diversify your diet, and not just consume mostly protein or completely eliminate carbohydrates from your diet. Don't be afraid to eat vegetables, fruits, nuts, fish, drink natural juices or water with a high mineral count, such as sodium potassium and magnesium. To lose twenty-two pounds in three months you don't need knowledge about the so-called longevity diet, therefore, I omit many important details in this book. However, I wanted to draw your attention to this point: do not eat just anything to make sure the number of calories agrees with your plan. Of course, you could arrange your diet so that you only eat two doughnuts and drink two quarts of cola each day, and you will certainly lose weight, but I am asking you to use a little common sense. Everybody knows that in the long run eating such things is not a healthy diet for anyone.

3.4. How many meals a day should I eat?

The recommended number of meals to be consumed each day remains a controversial topic. Some say five, while others say three meals are best. I recommend that you try out different options for yourself, adjust them to your own lifestyle, and stick to what works best and what you feel most satisfied with. Remember that not every person has the opportunity to eat five meals a day. Diet is only part of life and not the most important thing there is.

3.5. An example diet plan

Here are a few examples from my diet plan, illustrating the process of how my diet was gradually modified. Most importantly, I ate what I wanted, I was my own dietitian, and the weight was going down.

Before

- In the morning: coffee + sandwich.
- Around noon: lunch ordered at work, usually pizza or a piece of grilled chicken.
- At 5 p.m. dinner: vegetables + a piece of meat (fried with batter).
- At 9 p.m. supper: four sausage sandwiches.

In total I was eating about 3,100 calories per day. My first step was to lower the number of calories I ate for supper.

Week 1

- In the morning: coffee + sandwich.
- Around noon: lunch ordered at work—pizza or a piece of grilled chicken.
- At 5 p.m. dinner: vegetables + a piece of meat (fried in batter).
- At 9 p.m. supper: three sausage sandwiches.

Week 2

- In the morning: coffee + sandwich.
- Around noon: lunch ordered at work—pizza or a piece of grilled chicken.
- At 5 p.m. dinner: vegetables + a piece of meat (fried in batter).
- At 9 p.m. supper: two sausage sandwiches.

Week 3

- In the morning: coffee + sandwich.
- Around noon: lunch ordered at work—pizza or a piece of grilled chicken.
- At 5 p.m. dinner: vegetables + a piece of meat (fried in batter).
- At 9 p.m. supper: one sausage sandwich.

Next, I decided that my meal with the most calories was lunch at work, and I decided to change something there. I began to eat pizza only once a week, on Fridays. On other days, I brought my own lunch from home and only ate vegetables, lean meat, or fish, lots of spices, rice, or buckwheat.

Week 4

- In the morning: coffee + sandwich.
- Around noon: homemade lunch of lean meat or fish + rice or buckwheat + vegetables.
- At 5 p.m. dinner: vegetables + a piece of meat (fried in batter).
- At 9 p.m. supper: one sausage sandwich.

The next week I replaced my morning sandwich with a delicious shake that I prepared by myself. Typically, it was made with yogurt, banana, and blueberries, or yogurt plus strawberries.

Week 5

- In the morning: natural yogurt shake with fruit.
- Around noon: homemade lunch of lean meat or fish + rice or buckwheat + vegetables.
- At 5 p.m. dinner: vegetables + a piece of meat (fried in batter).
- At 9 p.m. supper: one sausage sandwich.

I made the next changes in the third meal of the day, which was dinner. I limited the number of dishes with flour to a minimum and gave up frying the meat in batter, instead I covered the meat with spices. I replaced my supper sausage sandwich with a sandwich made of turkey, tomato, cucumber, and paprika.

Week 6

- In the morning: natural yogurt shake with fruit.
- Around noon: homemade lunch of lean meat or fish + rice or buckwheat + vegetables.
- At 5 p.m. dinner: vegetables + a piece of meat (with spices).
- At 9 p.m. supper: one sandwich with turkey, tomato, cucumber, and paprika.

By gradually modifying my diet and decreasing in a simple way the number of calories I consumed by reducing the size of meals and their caloric content, while at the same time maintaining the tastes I enjoy, caused me to drop my weight from 190 pounds to 180 pounds in six weeks. According to my not-so-precise calculations, at the beginning I was eating about 3,100 calories per day, while after six weeks of gradually modifying my diet I consumed about 2,700 calories per day.

Over the next six weeks I continued to slowly modify my diet while using a little common sense. According to my calculations, I then lowered my intake to around 2,500 calories per day, and my body reacted to this by dropping to 168 pounds. I probably made a few small mistakes in my calculations, but one thing is certain: I controlled what I was eating and controlled my weight, and the entire time I felt happy and proud of my progress. At the same time, I did not have any feelings of regret from denying myself anything. Actually, I did not deny myself anything, but just the opposite. I replaced high-calorie food with meals with fewer calories that were still tasty.

3.6. How to end your slimming diet

To return to an optimal caloric balance (zero), you must not eat too few or too many calories. Therefore, if your weight has stopped at the level you previously chose as a goal, do not reduce or increase the number of calories in your diet and enjoy what you have achieved on your own. To find a golden balance can seem more difficult than it really is. In fact, weight measurements and the graph are more helpful at the end of weight loss than the beginning. Weight control is what allows you to maintain the same body weight for years, and any ups or downs will be quickly detected. Most importantly, you already know how to react when it happens.

4. What distinguishes my method from others?

With the Simple Weight Loss System™, you do not need to calculate your caloric need. Then why should you make these complicated calculations? It is enough to estimate the current number of calories you consume per day and reduce it at your own discretion, controlling your weight and what you eat on your own. The most important thing is that your weight drops; the exact amount of your caloric need is information that is actually irrelevant to you.

5. Overweight or obese?

If the weight of your body is slightly more than normal, we are talking about being overweight. In this case, the use of a simple diet you make yourself, such as with the Simple Weight Loss System™, is more than enough. Obesity means that the weight of your body is way above normal. In this case, the Simple Weight Loss System™ will also definitely give you the desired results, and it's worth to start reducing your caloric intake today. However, the difference between obese people and people who are overweight is significant, and I think that obese people should consult a specialist in order to have themselves examined and get a proper diagnosis. Very high body weight adversely affects your joints, your insides, and heart. After going above a certain weight, you must start taking your health seriously.

6. Problems you might encounter

6.1. Your social environment

One of the most difficult problems to overcome is your social environment. If you are currently in a situation in which greasy foods and sweet drinks are commonly served, you have a difficult road ahead of you. If your family, parents, siblings, or spouse eat large portions and serve high-calorie meals and you try to eat differently while living with them, it will not always be easy. If your colleagues at work order pizza every day, it can be difficult for you to not join them. You must be aware that this could be a problem, and you may have to face it if you decide to get rid of excess body fat. The good news is that you are not the only one who has this problem, as many people face the same difficulty and experience the same things you have to face. It is very difficult to break the standard routine and be different when everyone around you likes to eat a lot.

I will be straightforward—in such situations, you're on your own. I cannot tell you what you should do, because it will ultimately be your own choice. All I can do is share with you my experience. When I started to change my diet, at home everyone else ate differently, so I was forced to prepare my own meals separately, and I did. To my surprise, after some time, my family began to copy my dishes. Perhaps the visible effects caused them to start doing what I did, or they became motivated thinking "If it is working for him, I want to do it too," or maybe my food just tasted better. I do not know what caused this, but you can be sure that not only the environment you are in affects you, but you also affect your environment. Don't expect those around you to be willing to make changes right away as you have done, but after a while you may be surprised how big an influence you have had on them.

6.2. Loss of motivation

Motivation that disappears quickly is another problem that will keep you from reaching your goal. You have given yourself three months to modify your diet to lose as much as twenty-two pounds of fat, and you want to quit after only two weeks? You are not the only one who encounters this problem. It is something that happens to everyone because we are only human and we all have our moments of weakness. If your initial motivation is really strong and comes from you, you will certainly be able to make it through this temporary crisis. A decrease in motivation is not the end of the world, it is only a temporary crisis; and to achieve your goal you need to find a way to recharge your battery. Take a good look at your BEFORE picture and think about whether you want your AFTER picture to look the same or not? Read about how to deal with loss of motivation. Watch videos on the internet of people who managed to lose weight and who share their stories. Motivation is like a camp fire, you have to toss more wood on the fire from time to time to keep it burning.

6.3. Lack of ideas for new dishes

Are you at a loss of ideas for new tasty dishes, and the thought of grilled chicken with rice and vegetables is not appealing? Remember, you are not the only one with this problem. Fortunately, there are many recipes in books, on the internet, and featured in culinary programs. All you need to do is look at the first food blog that you come across to find something inspiring. Look for one of the fitness video channels because they often really have great ideas for delicious dishes with low-calorie content. I too became tired of my new diet and did not know what to eat. I found a bodybuilder on the internet who was quite funny and recorded a series of cooking videos. Watching one of his videos, I almost cried with laughter when he took his enormous hands and peeled small potatoes and cut them into cubes. Later, I decided to try one of his dishes—minced meat with dried tomatoes in mustard sauce baked in the oven with potatoes. I was so surprised, as this dish tasted so good I felt like a little kid who was eating a lollipop for the first time in their life.

6.4. Diet (light) products

You need to be careful when modifying your diet. One of the pitfalls that you can easily fall into are diet or "light" products. I remember deciding to replace my ordinary cornflakes with "light" flakes without checking the ingredients on the back of the package. I poured a handful of flakes into a bowl of milk, and when I started to eat them I was in shock because it was so sweet! I checked the ingredients, and it turned out that the "light" flakes contained additional amounts of sugar. I could not believe that this so-called diet product contains more calories than its usual equivalent. However, the food industry goes by its own rules. As a consumer trying to get rid of a lot of fat from your body, you must be especially attentive when buying different products such as yogurt or a snack bar labeled as "fit," "diet," or "light." In many cases these products contain added sugar. Remember, especially when buying a product for the first time, carefully check the ingredients listed on the packaging.

6.5. Insufficient water intake

Adults should drink an average of about two and a half quarts of fluids a day. Providing the right amount of water to your body is very important, and especially to lose weight. Insufficient water intake can slow down the whole process, because water is the main component of our bodies. To recognize if you have a water shortage, simply evaluate the color of your urine. If your urine is a pale straw color, you have perfect water management. If your urine is dark yellow, it means you lack water. Be sure to drink enough water every day, and you will soon see the wonderful effect of water on your body as it cleanses it from various toxins.

6.6. Lack of support

It is no secret that going through a long and tedious weight loss process is not an easy task for some. If you are alone and have no one to offer you support, look for a friend or colleague who is also interested in losing unnecessary pounds. If none of your friends wants to lose weight, find a diet buddy on a dieting or fitness website. Just keep searching until you find someone. If the other person is going through the same thing you are, it is much easier to understand and support each other. When you go through a weak period, your friend supports you, and vice versa when they want to give up you support them. On top of that, the common topic of diet connects you, and you can discuss things together, share positive and negative experiences, exchange ideas for new dishes, and so on. When you have the same goal as someone else, it makes it easier to reach it. If you do not have a sparring partner for weight loss, and the lack of support is bothering you, do your best to find such a person as soon as possible.

7. How to gain weight?

When emaciated people come to me, they often ask, "I would like to put on weight, can you help me?" I present them with my Simple Weight Loss System™. These people are shocked: "Are you nuts! Do you want me to weigh even less than I do now?" I answer that this system can be used not only for weight loss but also for weight gain. Familiarize yourself with it, and instead of reducing the number of calories you consume each day, increase them gradually—about 100 to 200 calories per day for a good start and be sure to keep an eye on your weight.

8. The Simple Weight Loss System™ in a nutshell

1. Get motivated, then take a BEFORE picture.
2. Weigh yourself.
3. Determine your goal: how many pounds and in how many weeks you want to lose them.
4. Have a notebook in which you record your weight regularly (weekly).
5. In the notebook, write down your current diet and calculate exactly the number of calories there are in each meal.
6. Modify your diet at your own discretion, keeping in mind that you only want to minimize the number of calories consumed per day.
7. Observe the chart of your weight. If after two weeks your weight does not drop, then modify your diet again by decreasing the number of calories consumed by another 100 to 200 calories per day.
8. Take small steps toward your goal and be proud that you are doing it.
9. After reaching your goal, it is time for a reward. Take an AFTER picture and compare it with your BEFORE picture.
10. Keeping your weight at the right level should not be a problem because you compose your own diet yourself, which means that you continue eating the things you like the most. The only difference is that you consume fewer calories per day than you did previously.

Conclusion

I was shocked when I first found out for myself that the Simple Weight Loss System™ works. Then three more times I have used this method to not only slim down but gain weight when I started to practice amateur powerlifting. Nutritional counseling has become my great passion after work hours, and now I willingly help hardworking people like myself deal with unnecessary weight. My simple method of weight loss has proven extremely effective, and in each case gives the desired results. Only customers who gave up after a couple of days did not have the opportunity to find out for themselves that it works. Instead, they chose to try chemical fat burners, and when those didn't work they decided there was no help for them. Dear reader, if you really want to get rid of unnecessary pounds, take another look at my BEFORE and AFTER pictures, and then find out for yourself.

Samuel F. Valle

This book is not enough for you, and you want to increase your knowledge? I highly recommend you to read the book "The JUST CUT IT™ method" by Jennifer Morris.

www.ingramcontent.com/pod-product-compliance
Lightning Source LLC
Chambersburg PA
CBHW041227270326
41934CB00004B/192